1

Man-Opause™
My Continuing Battle with Metastatic Prostate Cancer

by Gary Harris

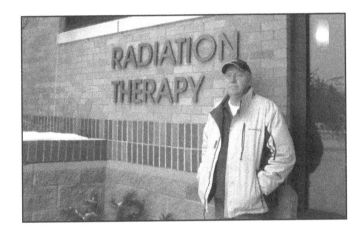

First Edition   ISBN: 978-0-578-54064-1

Happy are those who remain faithful under trials, because when they succeed in passing such a test, they will receive as their reward the life which God has promised to those who love him.

James 1:12 GNTD

This book is dedicated to those that have fought prostate cancer and lost, medical professionals that are focused on innovative, cutting edge research and healing, my family and friends that have provided unfailing encouragement and support both in thought and deed and in the power of our faith in God that provides the ultimate strength to fight and succeed in conquering cancer.

Credits

Cover design by Marc Harris, www.mvhart.com

Photos Mark Fallen, M.D., & Walter Roberts, M.D.,Ph.D with permission

All photographs by Gary & Sharon Harris

Special thanks to Dutch & Irma Cragun, Carl Boberg & Ann Hutchings for initial publication support

Contents

Foreward

From the first pages of "Man - Opause" you will be treated to very intimate experiences with husband, father, community volunteer, retired businessman and Land Surveyor Gary Harris. You will share his early fears of the unknown enemy; Recurrent Metastatic Prostate Cancer.

Gary takes you on his "homework and research trail" which made him victorious. Eleven years brought with it four separate diagnosis of prostate cancer including tumors and bone cancers followed by many scans, biopsies, surgery, radiation and chemotherapy and he has survived and won!

This inspirational book is essential reading as Gary shares his logical and spiritual decisions with you. He credits his wife Sharon, family, friends and faith in God for his remarkable recovery. The combination has produced a joyful, positive, active man anxious to praise his providers and share his story with you.

Please read and join Gary through his ordeals and triumphs as he begins a new phase with the formation of his prostate cancer support group to share information about the disease and its affect on men and their families.

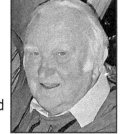

Merrill (Dutch) Cragun

"Welcome to Retirement"

prologue

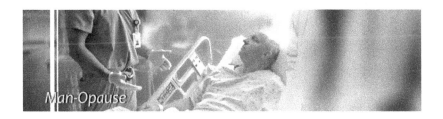

Man-Opause My Continuing Battle with Metastatic Prostate Cancer

It was spring 2008 and Cousin Al's 80th birthday celebration in St. Cloud Minnesota when my cell rang. I hesitated and answered only to hear "Gary, this is Dr. Fallen calling". I excused myself from the table, went to another room and offered a cordial "hi", knowing full well that this call will probably change my life as I knew it forever.

I had just retired from 40 plus years as a Licensed Land Surveyor and years of being owner or manager of civil engineering and land surveying firms in the Twin Cities. We had recently moved from the south suburbs of Minneapolis to our newly remodeled home in the lakes area of northern Minnesota near Brainerd. My wife Sharon and I were looking forward to great years together on the lake, golfing and enjoying retirement with longtime friends. We had visited the area regularly over the last several decades and were fortunate to have a family summer cabin on Clark Lake near Nisswa. Relocating from Minneapolis after 65 was to be a wonderful change in lifestyle.

"I have the test results from your biopsies and it is cancer".

Dr. Mark Fallen, M.D. one of the area's top urologists and surgeons was the one I turned to after a routine annual physical examination by my family physician and the discovery of a lump on my prostate gland. Dr. Fallen went on, *"I have the test results from your biopsies and it is cancer"*. I truly was not surprised but my knees began to buckle, my heart raced and my palms began to sweat as I fought my expanding emotions. My initial thought was that coming from a family history of heart disease and some of my own as a young man, I expected a heart attack would get me first, not cancer. I was totally unprepared for this. He continued, *"of the eleven biopsies we took, just one came back positive and tested medium in grade"*. This seemed at the time to be the good following the bad news.

We agreed to sit down in a few days to discuss the available treatment options that were open to us and the call ended. I tried to catch my breath and composure convincing myself that I could return to the table and keep this to myself so as not to damper the upbeat birthday feelings in the room.

I walked into the room and immediately felt the eyes of most at the table, who were somewhat aware of my possible diagnosis. It became quickly evident that putting up a false front and getting through the next few minutes, much less another hour or two, was a virtual impossibility. Sharon, my wife of 40 years at the time, was extremely anxious as her fear was that the worse was about to happen while still holding hope and praying that all would be good. She was pleading with her eyes to know the results of the call and most of the others were also hanging on to the same thread.

Unfortunately, I failed miserably . . . . . tears welled up in my eyes as I let the news out and I realized that I had just dropped a very large wet blanket on Al's celebration and dinner. He seemed oblivious to what was happening as he was somewhat hard of hearing and thankfully was not affected by my news. My mind has apparently blocked out the most of the rest of the day as I was struggling with Dr. Fallen's words and trying to come to grips with the "Big C" which was now an integral part of our lives.

If at the time, some ten years ago, I had any comprehension of the battles to be fought in the future for Sharon and myself, I wonder if the fears may have been insurmountable and depression would also have been an enemy to contend with. But we had no idea of

". . . . . . . .there were few words needed."

what lay around the corner in the years to come as prostate cancer has revisited on four occasions in varying degrees of severity since the initial surgery in 2008.

It was a long, quiet drive back to Brainerd that afternoon. We were concerned solely with the here and now and struggling with the problem of what we should be saying to each other. As soul mates however, there were few words were needed.

I am a Christian and have been a believer in God, Jesus Christ and the Bible for many years but it pales in comparison to that of my life partner Sharon. She has a very sacred connection with her God and faith and I thank her for her presence in my life and for orchestrating God's hand in our decisions and treatments over the last ten plus years. This relationship between Sharon and God has ultimately brought me closer as well and my life has been forever changed because of it.

Life and its battles require a team to be positive and inquisitive and I have been fortunate to have been surrounded with many loved ones, great friends and wise, well trained and highly motivated medical experts.

My goal in writing this account of my battle with metastatic prostate cancer is not to just to revel in the achievements of the medical community and how diligent and blessed we have been, but to inform and arm others with information and tactics to wage an even more effective battle by understanding this disease, minimize errors in judgment and the importance of placing unwavering faith in your family, friends, medical experts and a higher authority.

As you read my story, please remember that I am not trained nor in the business of medical treatment, but a patient like many others and, a triumphant survivor to date despite the long adds against me.

The fight has been long and difficult but I have been blessed big time.

In a nutshell, over the last ten years I have undergone surgery for a radical prostatectomy to remove a cancerous prostate and thirteen lymph nodes; radiation treatment for a recurrent prostate cancer tumor adjacent to my bladder; chemohormonal infusion therapy (chemotherapy) for recurrent prostate cancer lesions in two ribs, two locations in my spine and my sacrum (tail bone); radiation therapy for a recurrent prostate cancer tumor in my lower pelvic area; targeted high dose radiation therapy in all of the bone lesion areas previously treated with chemotherapy; and some twenty plus scans, most of which have occurred within the last eight years.

I may have made what now appear to be decisional errors, but in retrospect I would probably make again as they appeared to be logical, based on solid research, expert opinion and a seemingly good gamble at the time.

I trust the reader will benefit from this effort but bear in mind that all of life is a gamble based on our daily decisions with most being relatively inconsequential as compared to a life battle. When it comes to health decisions, we need to be positive, rely on research, testimony, recommendations from highly trained and experienced experts and loving support from others and prayer.

" The ultimate decision is always yours ...."

You must keep in mind that professionals in any field are human and subject to their own preferences, biases, and beliefs. The ultimate decision is always yours to discover the correct path of action, as well as the consequences.

An informed patient is a smart patient and with prostate cancer, one needs to work at completing a jigsaw puzzle where every individual piece is another bit of information that ultimately will form a picture of your overall health.

Assembling these puzzle pieces takes part over decades beginning in a man's forties and begin with regular physical exams that consist of, but not limited to, a digit test of the prostate by an experienced MD, a Prostate Specific Antigen (PSA) test, and a discussion of urinary problems, if any. None of these items by themselves will lead you to a diagnosis but in aggregate begin to tell a story. They are stepping stones that when placed correctly will lead you toward continued health or indicate additional testing to discover the existence of a cancer and its degree of severity.

As in the vast majority of cancers, early discovery is the most important factor in avoiding metastasizing of cancer and ultimately controlling or eliminating it. On the flip side of the coin, if cancer has taken the next step and has become a part of your being, moving ahead in an informed and logical way and remaining positive in your faith and support team will greatly increase your odds of survival and success in the days ahead.

My faith has been rewarded with at least one great miracle in the past several years and we are thankful for it. Are we entitled to another? Only time will tell. There was a period in my life when miracles were not preeminent but neither was my faith in God. Through the years, this has changed as my belief in the power of Jesus Christ has grown to the point where I now firmly believe success is accomplished with the power of prayer.

To date God has healed and spared me for a reason but until recently the path was unknown to me. My writing of this memoir of my battle with spreading proslate cancer is the beginning of my reaching out to others and fulfillment by paying back, in part, for my blessings. By doing so, my aim is to help avoid a life threatening advance of the disease in others through early screening and detection and the sharing the importance of assembling a trusted and experienced team when treatment is required.

"The Discovery"

Chapter 1

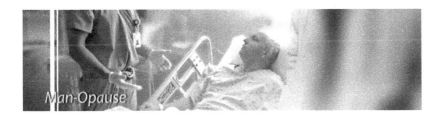

Man-Opause

It may sound strange, but I can not remember experiencing symptoms of my prostate cancer during any of its occurrences to date or prior to the original diagnosis in 2008. It seems to have been a silent disease that was sneaking up on me and by the time symptoms had become evident, it may very well have been too late.

I cannot count the number of times I have thanked my family physician for having the experience and expertise to locate a lump on one side of my prostate during an annual physical examination. This digit test usually took less than five or ten seconds when dealing with a normal shaped and sized prostate gland. I noted that on this particular occasion it was taking considerably longer and I asked if he had found something unusual. He assured me that he indeed found a lump and at that point I noted another "lump" in my throat as well. A PSA test was then ordered to add a second piece to the puzzle and the tests revealed an elevated reading of 5.6, considerably above a normal healthy prostate of approximately 3.0 nor less.

As I noted previously, cancer diagnosis becomes a series of puzzle pieces that ultimately produce an image from which an informed opinion can be formulated. Neither the digit exam nor PSA test is indicative of prostate cancer in their own right, but are facts that point you to the next step in the process.

This was exactly my case and fortunately I knew where to turn - that was Dr. Mark Fallen. He agreed to see me within the next few days and performed a second PSA test, which confirmed the results of the first. Another puzzle piece was formed. Dr. Fallen set up an appointment about a week later to perform biopsy tests of the prostate and the associated lump.

The biopsy is a tissue sample of the gland that is taken utilizing ultrasound or magnetic resonance imaging (MRI) for guidance and spring-driven needle core biopsy device (biopsy gun). Access to the prostate is through the lower colon. These are tissue samples taken randomly across the prostate and may or may not reflect the true degree of cancer as the more serious locations may have been missed in the sampling. Generally, between 11 and 15 samples are obtained. I found this process to be somewhat *"It was a sobering meeting."* uncomfortable but a necessity so I perservered through eleven samples. The tissue samples were then submitted to a laboratory for testing and Gleason Score grading (details later in this chapter) in the event cancer was detected.

Within a few days of the infamous dinner party call from Dr. Fallen, we met at his office for a strategy session and a discussion of the alternatives open to us. It was a sobering meeting. The three of us had grown to be quite comfortable with each other as Dr. Fallen had worked diligently several years before dealing with Sharon's struggle with kidney cancer which had a very successful and gratifying conclusion. His bedside manner of directness and caring definitely was fully engaged in our best care.

We discussed radical prostatectomy surgery (removal), radiation therapy, implanted radioactive seed therapy, cryogenics which was just coming onto the scene, hormone therapy, and simply monitoring and watching for progression. The latter has been somewhat common in men with a suspected low to medium grade of prostate cancer and especially those over 75 years of age, as the cancer could have relatively slow growth and not be as problematic as other age-related diseases might be.

I remember hearing more than once over the years that *"if you are going to get cancer, prostate is the one to get"*. Most men, assuming you live long enough, will be affected by it and many times causes only minor concerns. I personally believe this is somewhat blind to the facts, as even if your diagnosis indicates your prostate cancer is not serious at the onset, the situation can change dramatically.

Dr. Fallen recommended that the best place for my prostate and the cancer was *"in that stainless steel can in the corner of the operating room"*. Not hard to figure out what where he was heading. Again, he seemed not terribly concerned about speed due to the medium grade results of the biopsy and by this time it was June. I was thoroughly researching the different therapies available to me and the long-term odds of each; schedules with hospital surgery center; my being in the middle of a project or two and the availability of Dr. Fallen as he was the only person I would choose to do the surgery.

At the time of my surgery some eleven years ago, my surgery choices were the relatively new robotic method or standard open cut surgery. I had read about some negative results from robotics with errors being introduced by the machine operators and weighing that against the hundreds or thousands of standard surgeries that Dr. Fallen had done before, all with positive outcomes. I made the decision to go with him as this would also allow him to examine the entire pelvic cavity when excising the infected prostate. As a bonus this also allowed the repair of an existing hernia which was discovered at the time.

Prostatectomy surgery can leave some men impotent without successful nerve-sparing surgery resulting in a less than fulfilling sex life. I had placed my faith in Dr. Fallen to succeed in this aspect of the surgery. As for incontinence, sphincters get damaged in surgery either as a matter of necessity to eliminate cancer or mistakes due to human error, but I had "the best" and we moved ahead with a September 26th surgery date in Minneapolis.

I was quite confident and relaxed over the summer in the decision knowing full well that all of the options were investigated thoroughly

"I had no reason to be overly concerned ...."

and narrowed down to the chosen open surgery solution with Dr. Fallen and one of the best surgical hospitals in the Midwest. Of course, one always has the reality during the wait for surgery that I was walking and living with cancer and whether you acknowledge it or not, this does weigh on you emotionally. I had no reason to be overly concerned as we believed we were dealing with a normal, medium grade prostate cancer and it would shortly be eliminated. I was more concerned with the possible side effects from the surgery and their impact on our personal lives due to incontinence and/or impotence but again, my faith in the hands of Dr. Fallen kept me from dwelling on that aspect.

I continued to research the basics regarding prostate cancer and what it is. According to Dr. Pamela Ellsworth in her book 100 Questions & Answers About Prostate Cancer, Third Addition, some type of cancer will impact approximately 50% of men in the United States with the largest percentage of these being prostate cancer with the exception of skin cancers. Unfortunately, as of 2011, it was the second leading cause of cancer deaths in men. The good news is that these numbers have been dropping in recent years from increased awareness of the disease, improved diagnosis, and effective treatments. It is certain this trend will continue.

The Merriam Webster dictionary definition of cancer is "a malignant tumor of potentially unlimited growth that expands locally by invasion and systemically by metastasis". The definition of the prostate gland is "an organ found in men and male animals that produces the liquid in which sperm is carried". Accordingly, prostate cancer is the infection of the prostate gland by cells that are replaced uncontrollably and become what is commonly termed a tumor. Metastasis is described as "the spread of a disease-producing agency (such as cancer cells) from the initial or primary site of disease to another part of the body".

Thus metastatic prostate cancer is a cancer that has escaped the prostate gland and entered other surrounding tissues and/or the bloodstream. Both of these circumstances have been the foundation of my personal fight since the original surgery.

Prostate cancer is very closely related to sex hormones and very rarely develops in men that have undergone castration (ouch) early in life, but this is not common in the United States and certainly not in my world. Perhaps this is one reason that prostate cancer is much more prevalent in North America, Northern & Western Europe, and Australia/New Zealand than the rest of the world resulting in higher levels of testosterone which can increase risk of prostate cancer as prostate cancer thrives on testosterone. I view with concern the multitude of ads in print, television and the internet promoting testosterone boosting substances with very few warnings of the increased risk of growth of existing prostate cancer. Especially with those men that have undetected cancer in their systems the increased testosterone levels will have a marked increase in the growth of prostate cancer.

As men age the amounts of testosterone in their systems decrease while at the same time the odds of prostate cancer rises dramatically. Adding testosterone could be lethal if caution and testing prior to the addition of boosters to your diet is not a part of your overall health plan.

Grading of cancers is a very technical subject and I am not about to tackle it in depth with this book but there are excellent publications available that explain this in detail. In my case, Dr. Fallen preferred to talk in terms of Gleason scores rather than stages as after the surgery was completed and the pathology reports of the removed prostate were given to him, the degree of cancer found was now a known quantity. Gleason scoring has changed since 2008 and since 2018 the scores are now called Grade Groups. The new system is slowly being adhered to as the older system is being phased out. At the date of my surgery the scoring was as follows:

Gx: grade cannot be assessed

G1: Gleason score 2-4

G2: Gleason Score 5-6

G4: Gleason score 7-10

The scores are determined by testing of two main areas of cancer in the prostate and are calculated as 3+3=6;

3+4=7; or 4+3=7. The desired score, of course, would be the Gx as the cancer is very inactive and confined. A Gleason score of 7 or above can very threatening on the other side of the curve and is many times referred to as grade 5. My Gleason score was 3+4=7.

The new 2018 Grade Group scoring system is as follows:

Grade Group 1 = Gleason 6 (or less)

Grade Group 2 = Gleason 3+4=7

Grade Group 3 = Gleason 4+3=7

Grade Group 4 = Gleason 8

Grade Group 5 = Gleason 9-10

Prostate cancer screening is by far the best method to detect cancer early and catch it when it is "curable". Screening is best initiated with healthy men in their forties to 50 with those that have a family history of prostate cancer beginning at 40. The screening should consist of a digital rectal exam and a serum prostate specific antigen (PSA) test and be performed annually.

As previously discussed, PSA is not convincing evidence in its own right of cancer but simply a marker or puzzle piece to the overall picture. Some elevated PSA readings do not associate with cancer at all but a change in the scores should be watched carefully as this may be indicative of cancer growth.

Not all in the medical community subscribe to PSA testing as they feel that it may direct treatment and unnecessary worry to those that may have cancer that is undetectable to physical exams and may not cause an individual harm. Personally, I have some problem with moving through life without knowledge of how my family may be impacted by what is unknown today but may produce lethal consequences in the future.

I continue to spread the prostate cancer gospel to as many as I can to encourage all to be diligent in both physical examinations and PSA testing.

"The Ride Begins"

Chapter 2

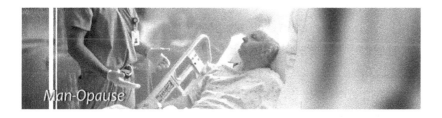

Man-Opause

Two days prior to surgery, our Pastor from The Journey Church Nisswa, Scott Pederson, paid us a visit for fellowship and prayer. We talked about the events ahead and the role that God, family, and friends played in them, especially the power of prayer and faith. Scott's closing prayer with us struck me as extremely optimistic as he prayed that the surgeon would find no cancer but in any case, I was in God's hands. How wonderful that was.

September 25, 2008, was upon us and surgery for the radical prostatectomy was scheduled for early the next morning in South Minneapolis. As we lived in northern Minnesota and it was required to be near the hospital the day before to prep for the road ahead including bowel cleansing, special liquid diet and rest. We are very fortunate in life to be blessed with very close and special friends that we have known and loved for several decades. The Nelson family, Bruce, and Kathy, were there for us and we drove to their Eagan (a suburb of Minneapolis) home. It was here that I was able to complete my preparation and be nurtured by the comfort of Sharon, Bruce and Kathy in an environment that was like home.

 In the late afternoon, dinner was being prepared (although mine was broth, Jell-O and water) when the front doorbell rang and there stood our daughter Joy and son Marc who had just flown in from San Diego and Arizona to be with us the following day. What a surprise, I was blown away by my family all being at my side and to this day will still bring a tear to my eyes. My loving wife

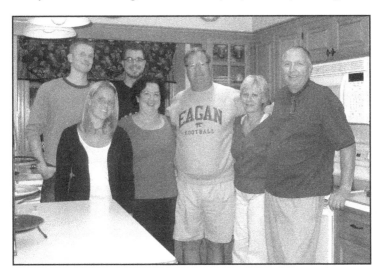

thought of everything! We all enjoyed a wonderful evening together and bright and early the next morning Bruce drove us to the hospital and we were off on an unknown merry-go-round ride that held many hidden surprises, both good and bad.

A week or so before, I had contacted a good friend, Pastor Dave Satre of our previous Burnsville, Minnesota church family, and asked if he would take the time on the morning of the 26th to be with Sharon, Joy, and Marc during my scheduled surgery. Without hesitation he was there and provided comfort and support for them during the long morning hours *"I was definitely comforted"* which to this day has been greatly appreciated.

I was in the best hands possible now with the best surgeon, hospital, staff, family, friends, and God all on my side. The last thing I remember prior to being wheeled to the operating room was hugging my family and Dr. Fallen came out to see me with a few relaxing words. I jokingly asked him if he was going to be careful. His response; *"I have never lost a sphincter and I'm not going to start with you"*. I was definitely comforted.

To this day I am not aware of the time that elapsed from beginning to end but for years I have listened to Sharon telling many people how the operating room was In constant communication with her. She swears that a nurse appeared and talked with them in the family lounge every 15 to 20 minutes giving a blow by blow description of the events in the operating room. . . . . . We were in the right place!

I awoke several hours later in the recovery room. Sharon,

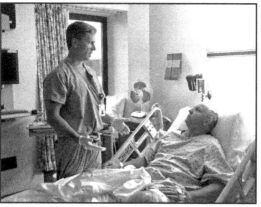 Joy, and Marc were there and I didn't have a clue which planet I was on, much less what was happening to me. Wires, hoses, a catheter, medication bags, beeping sounds, oxygen, nurses and everything else that goes along with

major surgery was about me but my most vivid memory was the awful taste in my mouth. Sometime later I was transferred to the surgery floor for constant monitoring with all of the appendages of the recovery room.

Between the painkillers, inability to move and a great deal of anesthesia remaining in my system, sleep came easy, other than being probed and prodded hour by hour by very professional and caring nurses aiding my recovery and verifying that I was still alive.

Dr. Fallen was one of the first to stop by the morning of the 27th to also verify that I made it. His bedside manner was much more serious than what I was used to in the past. He did first mention that he was able to spare both nerves that could cause impotence if damaged severely or cut despite one was very close to the actual tumor area. I was very relieved at this news and probably smiled broadly.

Sharon recalled that Dr. Fallen was pacing the room and clutching a small handwritten scratch note. He continued on that he had just picked up the pathology reports from the lab work on my prostate gland and the surrounding thirteen lymph nodes that he had removed during the surgery. I noticed that he had become somewhat pale in the face and proceeded to tell us that in spite of the original biopsies of June being positive in only one of eleven tissue samples, 25% of the prostate was cancerous and slightly less than 5% was grade 5, which may have been metastatic and spread to other areas or the bloodstream.

To say the least, the mood in the room changed very quickly from celebration and relief to confusion, trepidation, and fear. I swallowed hard and Sharon showed a flash of foreboding that scared me even more.

Dr. Fallen was quick to fill the emptiness in the room by explaining the depths that he went to in the operating room to carefully examine the prostate cavity and was reassuringly convinced that he *"got it all"*. Of course, there is an exception to every rule and statement and guarantees were impossible. I remember asking where we go from here and not concentrating on how this happened or *"why me?"*.

From day one I have been aware of the consequences and reality of cancer, but there were a few instances in which I did not believe we would be victorious.

"My New Best Friend Foley"

Chapter 3

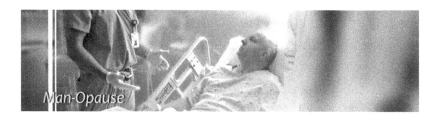

We spent the next three days and nights at the hospital gaining strength and ridding my body of what seemed like gallons of drugs and anesthetics. I had to learn to live with considerable pain and incapacitation as the decision to go with open cut surgery rather than robotic results in considerable damage to muscle and tissues that must heal and be rehabilitated. It was also necessary for me to get used to my new best friend for the next two weeks or so, the Foley catheter.

Dr. Fallen proclaimed that my main task for the next two weeks was to protect the cathcter at all costs, to keep it clean and free of crud and for heaven's sake, keep it in.

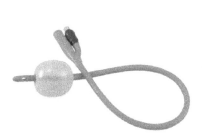

This thing was really uncomfortable. If you can imagine a quarter inch hose beginning in your bladder, traveling through your urethra, exiting down your leg and terminating in a plastic sack attached to your left ankle, you might understand.

The day bag was quite streamlined and somewhat inconspicuous other than the coiled hose in my shorts and the elastic strapping around the thigh that was intended to keep it all in place. Great theory but the reality was that it constantly worked itself down my leg as movement occurred resulting in extreme discomfort at the very point that the tube exited my torso. It took a few days, but I finally mastered the technique of utilizing good old fashioned duct tape to anchor the whole system to my thigh. Some degree of comfort was then achieved but the end of the two weeks could not come fast enough.

There was a benefit that I distinctly remember to old "Foley" and that was that you never felt the urge to visit a bathroom as the sphincter was disabled and drainage was allowed to occur steadily for the two weeks. However, you dare not forget to visit a men's room on occasion to drain the bag to avoid rupturing which could be somewhat embarrassing.

More than once I attracted some attention in public restrooms as I rested my foot on the edge of a toilet or the lip of a urinal, bent to lift my pant leg and popped the cork on the bag to relieve myself. Smiles were occasionally evident. The night bag was considerably larger, quite strong and allowed several hours of sleep before requiring service. When the time came to empty the bag, it was quite heavy and in my weakened state of recovery it was often necessary to drag my foot and leg to my destination but was always without incident.

During the surgery, drain tubes were installed in both the right and left sides of my abdomen to allow the fluids to escape that were accumulating internally from the healing process, and these were to be removed in a week or so or after the drainage ceased. To avoid having to make the

160 mile trip to Dr. Fallen's office just to have the drain tubes removed, my new internist, Dr. James Freeman, in Brainerd was kind enough to perform this task. He also performed the pre-surgery physical for me in early September which was my introduction to him culminating in our professional relationship becoming very close ever since.

"The main event was to have my buddy "foley" removed....."

My first return checkup with Dr. Fallen's office was about two weeks after surgery and the main event was to have my buddy "Foley" removed and be able to return to a somewhat normal lifestyle. To say the least, I was excited for this to occur. It was only a five-minute procedure and the last words of advice were something like *"if you don't urinate within five or six hours, get to an emergency room"*. These were not comforting words as I was sent out into the cold, cruel world but I thanked God as I had been rewarded with "Foley" being in the trash can instead of in me. Success was achieved a few hours later at the Nelson home as I was not about to hit the road for Brainerd until I knew all was working again. It was gratifying once again to actually feel that I had to relieve myself from time to time and my new best friend for a period of time was now "Depends ᵗᵐ".

It was also great to be free of the restrictions of tubes, tape, bags, drains from my prostate cavity and the end of sleeping in a lounge chair. The thought of actually sleeping in a bed was very exciting and I felt exhilarated although it may have been the end of peaceful nights for wife Sharon. The healing process went very well and I worked hard at strengthening my body back to its finely tuned sixty-six-year-old condition of pre-surgery days.

Dr. Fallen was concerned with the unexpected results of the post-surgery pathology reports wherein my return to his office in three months for an exam and the all-important first PSA test was constantly on our minds. As a reminder, PSA is the acronym for prostate specific antigen and a blood test score above zero indicates cancer in those that have had the prostate removed. Waiting three months for this test allows the body to rid itself of the pre-surgery PSA remaining in my system but some additional time may be required to give a complete answer. A decreasing score would at least indicate a trend in the right direction. As there was a possibility that the cancer already had metastasized and begun spreading to other areas of the body, this test was even more important that it has an outcome of being near zero.

All of life is a waiting game and this may have been the longest three months for us in many years, but our relationship with Jesus Christ, our God, great friends and the hundreds of prayers being said for us across the country made it easier to deal with on a daily basis.

On our drive to the office of Dr. Fallen in January, the mood was somber but hopeful for a positive result. His staff removed the required blood samples, sent them to the lab and I returned to the waiting room for the call to return for the results. After a short wait we were taken to an exam room where Dr. Fallen came in, without stopping for a breath and not being a melodramatic messenger of good or bad news, was wearing a grin and announced that my PSA was for all intents and purposes zero. Prior to this, Sharon was literally shaking and pale waiting for the results and watching that look change to one of exhilaration, relief and thankfulness was worth its weight in gold. Our trio was somewhat giddy as we were being rewarded for good deeds.

During the drive back to Brainerd we thanked our Lord and contacted Joy and Marc, some very special friends and relatives to share the good news with. They were very excited, happy calls and we could hear the relief in their voices with the great results. These people, among dozens more, were always there for us and shared in the stress and the celebration.

Fortunately, we had little idea at the time of what was around the corner for us. If we had any knowledge of the frustrations, battles, and victories in the years to come, it certainly would have burdened our hearts and minds.

"It Got Out"

Chapter 4

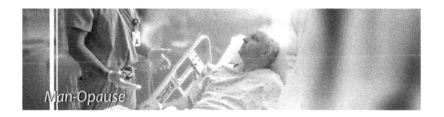

Man-Opause

Despite the elation of the moment, reality prevailed and the question arose as to where to go from here in order to manage my continued recovery and the possibility of cancer recurring in the future. The decision of deciding on a method of treatment of cancer, following through with it and then playing the waiting game over and over for results all go hand in hand. It would be grand to be able to say we have been victorious and can now walk away with few worries in the world. I personally know several men who have been fortunate to actually be in that position as their prostate cancer was either discovered and dealt with early or the severity of it was moderate to low and did not result in future recurrences.

As a result of the pathology report of the removed prostate, Dr. Fallen thought it best, despite his comfort level with our success, for us to consult with an

"We were both literally without words at this point ....."

oncologist at this point to discuss additional avenues of continued treatment for an overall, comprehensive approach to eliminating or at least minimizing the future consequences of the disease. His office set up an appointment for the consult with a local oncologist and we went to see him with some trepidation. This was a hard-hitting session and he had a no-nonsense approach to his profession recommending full treatments of chemotherapy, radiation and hormonal therapy. We were both literally without words at this point and it was a lot to struggle with after basking in our surgical success to date. But in retrospect, this was the point in time that a mistake may have occurred and a losing gamble taken. We opted for not proceeding with his recommended treatment regimen. In retrospect, moving on without following the recommendation of the oncologist may have proved to be the cause of some very tough times ahead, although the current practice in cases such as mine would be to watch and monitor. We decided along with Dr. Fallen to continue to carefully monitor, watch and wait as a three-month schedule was to be adhered to for PSA testing and annual digital examinations.

As a part of the prostatectomy surgery the nerve-sparing surgery was successful, but achieving erectile function was not expected for from twelve to twenty-four months as shock and partial damage to the nerves required time to heal and regain effectiveness. Incontinence during the next year was somewhat of a problem also, but again required time for the urethral sphincter and surrounding bladder control to regain a semblance of normal activity. For several months the rule of the day was don't wait when nature calls, and I didn't.

My next examinations at the six and nine-month intervals again resulted in PSA test scores of very near zero which brought about relief again and again. I was also happy that just prior to the nine-month test, life began once again in the land of the successfully spared nerves. This was exhilarating and ahead of schedule as we were not ready to pack that aspect of life in yet.

The next three-plus years drifted by with our stress levels growing every three months prior to spending a couple hours with our now very close friend and confidant Dr. Fallen. We thought we were not conscious of the stress levels building up to the PSA tests, but every time we were presented with the news that the result was zero we noticed a significant degree of relaxation on our drive back home. Not to worry, however, as it will happen once again at each three-month interval until we near the three-year point and then hopefully have the luxury of testing at six-month intervals.

More than three years was upon us and by this time the testing procedure and resulting zeros were getting to be somewhat anticipated. Dr. Fallen completed my annual physical exam which was without a problem while we awaited the lab results of the PSA blood draw. When he returned to the room he was not smiling and very seriously stated that the number was 0.07 instead of the 0.03 or less of previous tests (for all intents and purposes 0 was 0.03 or less). At first, this did not seem like a big deal to us but he went on to inform us that this most likely indicated that I had recurrent prostate cancer testing positive and it indeed metastasized some three years ago.

It got out! Our world was seemingly crumbling once again as the identity, degree and location of the cancer, of course, was unknown. Indeed -*"Where do we go from here?"*

An appointment was set up for a pelvic cavity ultrasound examination in Dr. Fallen's office to search for the culprit, which in all likelihood was a tumor or lymph node in the general area of the now non-existent prostate. This was a very interesting, but uncomfortable exam consisting of an ultrasound probe via the anal cavity that produced a picture of the pelvic area to the bladder.

I distinctly remember the doctor asking his assistant to hand to him an instrument, I recall being called "Gabriel's Horn".   Scary, considering the confined area that he was working in already was occupied by his hands and the ultrasound probe.

"I never did get a look at Gabriel's horn ...." I was fully awake and lying in a fetal position on my side and thought about inquiring what this new instrument was. After weighing the possible answers to my inquiry, however, I decided I really would be better off not having this knowledge and I just remained quiet and prayed for the best. I never did get a look at "Gabriel's Horn" or had the courage to investigate it. After being subjected to it I never wanted to hear the term again, at least not in proximity to my body. A tumor was found and Dr. Fallen's choice and recommendation for treatment was a Twin Cities based radiology clinic as he had a positive working

relationship with them over the years and had confidence in their work.

To my benefit, they had an office in Brainerd located in the St. Joseph's Hospital and Dr. Fallen concurred with the location choice as this was also near our home. The office was headed by Physicist and Radiation Oncologist Walter Roberts. MD, Ph.D. who had joined the firm following studies at the University of Michigan, Ann Arbor and Wayne State in Michigan.

I set up an interview with Dr. Roberts to determine his analysis of my problem and just as important to determine my comfort level with him, his staff and technology.

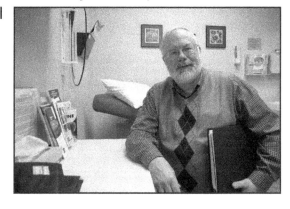

I reiterate that when selecting the professional team members that you research, check credentials and speak with others that were familiar with the individual and have recommendations based on experience. I was fortunate to have a very close friend who had recently completed treatment with Dr. Roberts for lung cancer and had a very positive recommendation for him and the clinic.

When you are confronted with a life and death option it is imperative that you work with the best in the field and with those that are confident in their ability. Dr. Roberts was warm and extremely well trained and learned in the fields of physics and radiology and I was convinced that he knew exactly where we were headed and that failure was not an option. It was also impressive that they had just finished installing and testing some five million dollars worth of the latest nuclear linear accelerator hardware to accurately pinpoint and target the tumor. Dr. Fallen had provided Dr. Roberts with the complete examination and ultrasound information from my last session with him and my past history of the disease, surgery, and testing.

Dr. Roberts completed MRI and CAT scans of their own and produced a plan of attack to eliminate the tumor with a regimen of thirty-three sessions of radiation therapy. They were to be daily with the exception of weekends and Holidays and to begin in the middle of November 2012 and end after the turn of the year. The staff was very conscientious and prided themselves on their professionalism. They precisely executed the treatment plan that Dr. Roberts developed for my treatment with permanent tattoo marks on my torso and prepared a body cast that would keep me aligned perfectly during the treatments for the short daily exposures over the next thirty-three sessions.

The holidays were approaching and the treatment schedule was a bit of an inconvenience but a necessity and we moved positively ahead. It also provided an opportunity for Joy and Marc when they visited for several days at Christmas, to experience this treatment up close and personal as the clinic allowed them access to one of my treatments and had the opportunity to have much of it explained by Dr. Robert's staff. I trust this intimate visit with my family may have been a bonding experience for us all.

As the treatment schedule advanced and we neared the end, the radiation began to accumulate in my system and my stamina and strength began to diminish. This actually did not begin until about the third or fourth week and was very noticeable by the fifth. At the conclusion of the thirty-three sessions Dr. Roberts, his staff and other patients in the radiology waiting room had become quite close to Sharon and I and moving on was sweet sorrow, as with most we would never cross paths again.   I should point out,
that the   *"My battle was not completed ...."*
treatments
to eradicate the discovered tumor were very successful and it was eliminated with a heartfelt thank you to all involved. I vowed to return to the clinic as a volunteer to other patients going through these treatments in the future but unknown to me, my battle was not completed and my volunteering was postponed.

Three months later we were at Dr. Fallen's office for yet another PSA test and digital examination. This was a follow up to the completed radiation therapy as well as getting back on track for standard quarterly testing. If the eradicated tumor had not been discovered, the interval of testing probably would have been expanded to six months by now but for the foreseeable future we were remaining at three. The results of the digit exam were negative and indeed the tumor was gone but the PSA had not zeroed out as hoped and was approximately 0.12 indicating that cancer was more than likely somewhere else and we needed to find a method of locating it as well. An outside possibility was that the PSA level was elevated prior to the radiation and simply took a while to dissipate, but this was not the case.

The discussion once again became quite serious as options were identified and quantified. Dr. Fallen began to talk about an experimental program to pinpoint the location of the recurrent metastatic prostate cancer. It was being developed at only one location in the United States and just so happened to be in our geographic area. He added that it was a project of a colleague from his days of urology residency, Dr. Q, (for purposes of this writing not his real name) who had been conducting research to discover a means of diagnosing and locating recurrent metastatic prostate cancer and facilitating accurate treatment of it.

The procedure, a choline PET scan was still in its experimental stage, but Dr. Fallen believed that I should consult with Dr. Q to examine the possibility of being included in a program to locate the spread of my cancer. A call was made to set up a consultation and my medical records, both from Dr. Fallen and Dr. Roberts were sent to Dr. Q. After multiple telephone interviews they agreed to an appointment for us to discuss the options and program details and it was set for February 2012.

I spoke with Dr. Q's assistants on several occasions regarding the timing and the testing. I was informed that the scan was currently experimental and had not yet been given approval by the FDA. Accordingly, the approximate cost of the scan was $9,000 and was not covered by insurance or Medicare as I was 69 years old at the time.

Sharon and I discussed this and without hesitation, we wished to move ahead as this may be a small price to pay for the discovery of a life-saving opportunity. We looked forward to the consultation and this was an exciting moment in time. It was also our first ever visit at a specialized clinic and it held hope for a continued and effective treatment of my recurrent prostate cancer that we feared was threatening to deliver me to my Maker.

"Anxiety Turns to Panic"

Chapter 5

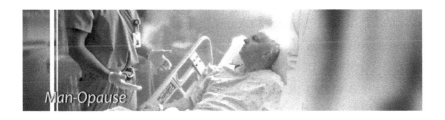

My PSA was 0.16 in February of 2012 and had been rising slowly for the past several months. This may seem like a low score but the fact that without a prostate it should have been very close to zero and it was moving upwards indicating that cancer was evident and growing. I was extremely pleased to discover that the scan may locate the position of recurrent cancer in my system and wanted to gather the information first hand from Dr. Q. This was the motivation behind my pressing for a consultation despite the PSA results not being at a recommended threshold of 1.0 or above to insure accurate test results.

In our meeting with Dr. Q that day, I clearly remember the statement that *"I was the healthiest patient in the clinic"* and I suspected that he may have been somewhat disturbed by the fact and that my visit was a waste of valuable time. As I discovered later in my experience with Dr. Q and his department, the bulk of his patients and their cancers were considerably more advanced than I was at the time, thus accounting for his analysis of my condition and less than urgent need for his services. Unknown to all of us at the time was that my condition was going to become very serious very soon.

I found him to be a very pleasant fellow and surrounds himself with assistants and staff that are as dedicated as he is. To show balance in his life, we were impressed that he also is a very talented musician and composer in his own right. I, on the other hand, am a "car guy", a photographer and have my guitar and banjo which provide my life balance.

The scan was explained in some detail to us temporarily solving my curiosity about it. Basically, choline, according to Wikipedia, is a water-soluble vitamin-Like essential nutrient found naturally in many common foods such as eggs, liver, beef, various vegetables, and breast milk. Over years of testing with many different substances and their relationship to prostate cancer cells, it was discovered that choline is readily absorbed by the cancer cells. When injected intravenously with glucose and a proper amount of a radioactive tracer followed by a combination PET and CT scan the result was the location of the errant prostate cancer cells. The scan must be completed within twenty minutes of the injection due to a radioactive half-life of the agent.

I do not wish to oversimplify this process, as it is highly scientific but the resulting scans, when read by experts, indicate prostate cancer as green colored areas on a computer monitor and is quite amazing to experience. The day will come in the next couple of years when I will discover just how amazing this tool really was. (for purposes of this work I will refer to this as "scan").

By November of 2013, my PSA scores had reached 0.84 and I once again contacted Dr. Q's office in December to inform them of this new elevated number in hopes of being able to schedule the scan. Again, they were recommending that my PSA be between 1.0 and 1.5 at a minimum to attain the desired level of accuracy in the test. To repeat, neither one of these numbers on the surface appear high until you take into account that when the prostate has been removed and you do not have prostate cancer it should be zero. Reluctantly, I agreed to continue the monitoring process and wait until it reached the requested levels.

I was beginning to feel like a walking Petri dish in that for the next year or so I had cancer growing inside of me seemingly unabated. The question being where is the cancer and what will be its effects on our lives? It was very difficult not to think about this alien within me on a 24/7 basis. My sleep was beginning to be affected, and my stress level was definitely beginning to show on an increasing basis. I was reminded more than once of the horror films where a monster bursts out of the torso of a victim. It is very hard to keep focused when you want to move ahead but we were delayed by circumstances beyond our control.

"....shows how fast things start to go wrong ......"

Cancer growth is geometric in that the cells replicate very quickly. An example is one becomes two, two become four, four become eight, eight then sixteen, sixteen becomes thirty two, etc. etc. until in a short period of time the cells number in the millions and the body's ability to fight it off begins to lose. My PSA score of 0.84 just a few months ago had now jumped to 4.6 in February of 2014!

Astonishingly, I was on a three-month interval for testing with Dr. Fallen which shows how fast things start to go wrong due to the out of control replication of cancer cells. Of course, we all became very alarmed and I made contact with Dr. Q and they immediately set up an appointment for the scan the second week in March. The waiting period for the scan is normally about three months and they apparently believed this was serious as well. I thought I was worried before, but now I was reaching new levels of anxiety, not to mention the impact it was having on my loving wife Sharon.

The scan was performed on March 17th along with an endorectal coil MRI. The latter is magnetic resonance imaging using an endorectal coil, a thin wire covered with a latex balloon that is inserted a short distance into the rectum. It provides images that are clearer and more detailed than other imaging methods. The results were discussed the next morning with Dr. Q and the images were viewed and reviewed in his office. The scan slices began at the skull and progressed through the body to mid-thigh.

I understood that metastatic prostate cancer has a history of settling in the ribs and there was some discussion in the viewing of progressive slices of the scan that a rib could be a location. Not surprisingly, this turned out to be the case as a telltale green glow appeared in two ribs along with two lymph nodes in the chest cavity. I noticed, however, that Dr. Q had an increasingly concerned look as significant evidence of cancer was found in my spine in two locations and my sacrum. Specifically, there were moderately intense lesions in the T12 and T8 regions of the spine and a markedly intense sacral (tailbone) lesion covering the entire tail bone.

I felt Sharon's grip on my arm intensify causing some pain as the events of the last four or five minutes set in and we both recognized that this was not your normal visit to the doctor's office. Dr. Q is a very cool guy but his mind had to be racing to catch up with the results, just as we were. How does he react so as not to send us into panic mode, but explain to us the serious nature of the situation, not that we hadn't already realized this?

".... he was shocked and commented that I should have been on morphine for the pain"

In my mind, this second recurrence of cancer, classified as #1 Metastatic Prostate Cancer, when compared to the initial pelvic cancer tumor, was like comparing a tornado to a rainfall. We had a lengthy discussion of the serious nature of the findings of the scan and treatments available to us, some better and most likely more effective than others. After noting the extent of cancer in my sacrum, Dr. Q asked me about the pain I must have been enduring. I responded that I had very little if any, and he was shocked and commented that I should have been on morphine for the pain in its present state. As for the lesions in my spine, I have considerable amounts of arthritis in my lower back being a more likely cause of pain and stiffness over the years than from cancer which may have accounted for my ignorance of cancer caused pain.

I wish to remind the reader here, that this may be a classic case of metastatic prostate cancer not always causing noticeable symptoms. Because of this, it is imperative to be proactive about monitoring your cancer and/or verifying its existence at all. To this day, I have no explanation for my lack of pain and symptoms throughout this war except by the hand of God.

We undertook the scans and testing hoping and praying for a relatively straightforward and much simpler diagnosis for the rising PSA levels of the last year and a half, perhaps just a rib or a lymph node or two. The actual diagnosis left us exhausted, confused and bewildered but I still can honestly state that we were positively looking for a solution and possible cure and not dwelling on *"why me"?* The reality is that using the term "cure" is more than one can expect with metastatic castration-resistant prostate cancer (mCRPC). Slowing the replication and production of cancer cells is currently the goal of today's treatments and NO DRUG has been developed to date that will kill all the cancer cells present.

I recall in our meeting to discuss the cancer diagnosis and possible remedies, that he mentioned a statistic that struck me as peculiar in that I fell in a class of clients where only 17% are as serious as mine. I wondered how he came up with such a precise number rather than a general number such as 20% and asked about it. He said the number was based on a known number of clients to date and the degree of their cancers. Still, I thought it strange but the elevated degree of concern was evident. The recommended therapy at this point was chemohormonal therapy rather than undergoing hormonal therapy or chemotherapy by themselves.

Dr. Q had a very close working relationship with an oncology clinic in the Twin Cities area and I was being referred to them to deal with my latest and very serious cancer discovery. Between them they had developed a regimen for docetaxel-based Taxotere tm, chemotherapy, a powerful drug developed from the

Intermittent Chemotherapy and Hormone Therapy

Day # 1 Taxotere infusion (75 mg/m²) + daily prednisone 5 mg BID—cycle 1

Day # 22 Taxotere infusion+ daily prednisone 5 mg BID—cycle 2

Day # 43 Taxotere infusion+ daily prednisone 5 mg BID—cycle 3

1-2 weeks post 3rd cycle, return to Mayo Clinic for restaging with C11 PET scan and get 1st Firmagon injection 240 mg
(May stop prednisone while on hormone therapy)
Also begin Casodex (bicalutamide) 50 mg daily while on Firmagon

28-30 days post 1st Firmagon—give 2nd Firmagon injection 80 mg
(Continue taking Casodex daily until chemotherapy is resumed)

28-30 days post 2nd Firmagon, begin Taxotere chemotherapy and prednisone BID x
Another 3 cycles—then restage with the C11 PET scan and back on Firmagon for 2 months.

European Yew tree that attacks prostate cancer cells and prevents or slows the cell division process.

This was to be administered intravenously (IV) on six occasions every three weeks at the oncology clinic along with the steroid prednisone to reduce side effects of fatigue, dry skin, nail deformation loss, and weight gain. The drug Zometa ᵗᵐ was also administered via IV along with the Taxotere ᵗᵐ to increase bone density due to bone loss from the cancer that was attacking my spine, ribs, and sacrum. It is also a preventative for osteoporosis. In my case, the cancer was attacking my bone density and Zometa ᵗᵐ replaced the lost calcium as the cancer cells were eliminated. Expected side effects of Zometa ᵗᵐ included constipation, bone pain, nausea, and weakness.

Prior to each chemo treatment, there was also administered by IV a nausea preventative which worked quite well as this was never a side effect of any of the treatments. It had its downside, however, and it wasn't until the third set of injections that I finally had a grip on severe constipation it caused and I countered it by taking large amounts of stool softeners and laxatives beginning a day or so prior to the chemo appointments.

After completing the first three rounds of chemo, a break of several weeks was prescribed and we returned to the care of Dr. Q for another scan to verify the interim success or failure of the chemotherapy. The results of the scan showed amazing improvement of the cancer lesions and provided evidence of bone locations that were actually being reclaimed with calcium. The improvement appeared to be in the range of 50% in the worst locations in the spine and sacrum with total remission in the ribs and lymph nodes at this half-way point of the chemotherapy. I also began hormonal therapy utilizing a new drug Firmagon ™ which was an alternative to the traditional Lupron ™ injections that have been used for a number of years. This is discussed additionally in Chapter 6.

I was told that some men have very few side effects from this chemotherapy regimen, however, in my case, this was not so. My normal routine was to feel quite good for three or four days after the injections and then be increasingly fatigued for the next ten or eleven days and then once again feel much improved for the last five leading up to the next chemo session and then repeat the process but with increasing difficulty. We were pretty good at adjusting our life cycles to coincide with the good days of the routine and avoiding a lot of social interaction during the low times. The fact that one might lose their hair as a side effect was very true with the drugs that were being administered and I was told that I would lose my hair in approximately 14 days after the first chemo session.

I carefully watched for adverse hair conditions and on the 14th night I washed my hair as always and not a hair was loose. I was becoming proud of my strong constitution and may prove hair loss to be an old wives tale. Early the next morning I woke Sharon and asked her to roll over as her hair was tickling my face as we slept. She responded that she was facing away and go back to sleep. To my shock, the itching on my face was in reality my own hair which fell out during the night and was scattered across my pillow. So much for my constitution! I paid a visit to my barber Ron that morning for a very close buzz cut. For several months I was complimented on a regular basis for having a head that was "made for bald", but it was cold.

The Hairball Incident: Between chemo sessions I had a tendency to feel quite good for several days following the infusions. This was followed by a period of fatigue and then I felt quite good again for a week or so leading up to the next session. We decided to fly to Denver to visit our son during one of these times and had a wonderful time with him and his cat Chloe. One evening I was sitting on the couch and Chloe had a habit of resting or sleeping on the top of the cushions and was doing so behind me. She began licking the top and back of my head for some reason and after several minutes of her rough textured tongue massaging my scalp I gently put an end to it.

In the middle of the night, I awoke and on my way to the bathroom I stepped on one of her hairballs on the floor. After close examination, I realized this was not cat hair but some of the remaining loose fuzz that she had removed my head. I stayed a safe distance from her for the next few days to avoid being the cause of her choking.

We discovered that the extended period of fatigue was caused mainly by dehydration as it is very difficult to orally ingest sufficient liquids to counteract the effects of the chemotherapy drugs. The dehydration and fatigue were so severe that on one occasion I passed out on the bathroom floor breaking my glasses and sustaining facial abrasions. By the fourth session in the second half of the program, the dehydration was countered with the cooperation of the oncology department at our local hospital and spending a few hours twice a week receiving an IV of fluids. This was like turning on a switch and temporarily relieved much of the fatigue that I had been experiencing.

Another important side effect of my chemotherapy was the loss and/or change in my taste sensitivity. In my case, it began within five days of the first session and lasted until three weeks or so after completion of the sixth session. I lost most of my taste for foods and liquids completely and found that sweets and sour foods were disgusting. One has to be careful when the loss of taste occurs as you lose your desire to eat and during chemo it is advisable to eat more than normal, not less. I found myself eating because I needed to, not because I wanted to and lost approximately fifteen pounds over the twenty plus weeks. There are better ways to diet.

Chemotherapy lowers the white blood cell count which in turn reduces your natural ability to fight infections and disease. To reduce this immune system failure a relatively new drug Neulasta ™ is prescribed by injection 24 hours after the chemotherapy session. An order was drafted by the oncologist for the Brainerd hospital's oncology department to provide the injections as this location was close to my home. The willingness of the hospital staff and their conscientious efforts when I needed them were appreciated. The development of this drug has brought with it an automatic injection system in 2018 that is installed on the patient's upper arm and is timed to inject the drug precisely 24 hours after it is activated thereby eliminating the return trip for the manual injection. This is a small point of truth that fighting hard for another day, week or month may bring about new technology and remedies to solve old problems as time passes.

Like most things in life, we learn by experience and by the time the chemo had come to an end, I had learned the ins and outs of the system and I trust that this will aid the reader if you or a loved one should ever have to go through similar treatment. I also found myself relying more and more on my faith, its wisdom and the Lord as a guide on a daily basis including the following passage from Psalms *"Love is demonstrated in magical ways."* 68:19 "Praise the Lord, who carries our burdens day after day; he is the God who saves us".

In a time of need, whether physical or emotional, God is our lasting crutch but people are amazing as they reach out to you in search of a way to ease your struggle. Close friends and relatives can strike a chord of comfort that remains with you well into the future. An example, Sharon's Sister Jan and husband Jack showed up one day for a visit and it happened to be on one of my especially low periods where the chemo had been hard on me. Jan hand knit a beautiful "Prayer Blanket" for me which has provided comfort for both Sharon and me to this date and in our home is never out of sight.

Love is demonstrated in magical ways.

"Man-Opause"

Chapter 6

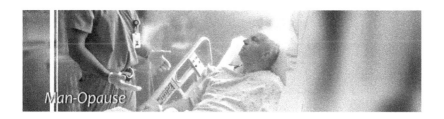

Hormonal therapy eliminates the production of testosterone by the testicles in effect starving the prostate cancer cells and reducing their ability to divide and spread. Hormone or androgen therapy is not a cure for prostate cancer, it simply reduces the activity of the cancer cells and slows production. The drugs Lupron™ and Firmagon™ both dramatically lower the amount of testosterone thereby eliminating libido, the ability to obtain erection, hot flashes resembling that of menopause in women and on occasion a few anatomy changes. Considering the alternatives, all were acceptable despite the discomfort and changes to our personal lives.

Herein lies the meaning behind the title for this writing "Man-Opause".   My wife Sharon is a very caring person, a wonderful partner and has been a caregiver throughout our married life. She does have a twisted sense of humor at times, however, and when the hot flashes began several years ago, she was quick to point out over and over that *now you know what I felt like*".

In response, I adopted the phrase "Man-Opause" as a defense mechanism and have used it over and over in conversations, with men and women. The term manopause was originally used by Time™ magazine in 2014 in an article dealing with low testosterone in men as a result of the aging process. Due to my treatment regimen I now have an understanding for the ladies that most men do not possess.

A year or two ago Sharon and I were flying to the west coast for a visit with our daughter Joy and I discovered an article in the onboard magazine discussing cancer and the side effects of chemotherapy. The term "chemo brain" was used to discuss changes in motor responses such as grip, random pains, neuropathy, clumsiness and the like that occur for many people in the months and years following the treatments. I too have experienced this as I have dropped and broken quite a few fragile dishes, dropped eating utensils, and threw Asian food at daughter Joy when my noodle filled chopsticks spun in my hands.

" ..... you're not as sharp as you used to be."

On occasion I have also been known to stumble and mutter uncontrollably.

There was a time in my life that I was quite agile, an athlete and fully in control but now Sharon has been heard to utter that "you're not as sharp as you used to be." At times this can be disconcerting, but considering the alternatives and that I now know the basis for some of my actions, not really a problem at all.

I received the Firmagon™ injections for three months when Dr. Q for multiple reasons, switched the therapy to Lupron ™, the original and older drug. The Firmagon™ was injected monthly into the stomach muscles one month on the left side and then alternating to the right side the next. The drug caused some very irritating side effects including a red very itchy and painful rash right where your belt line is. It also caused a very hard swollen area at the site of the injection that lasted for several weeks, all very irritating. Lupron™ is given by injection every three months rather than monthly and in the buttocks with relatively few, if any, of the painful and itchy side effects from the first drug.   Subsequent to the switch in drugs my only side effects in the ensuing years were those described at the beginning of this chapter including the infamous "Man-opause" hot flashes.

With renewed vigor and confidence that the chemotherapy and hormone treatments were actually defeating the cancer, the final three sessions of three-week infusions commenced. We encountered staffing at both the oncology clinic and the hospital to be very professional, caring and precise in their handling of patients and the sophisticated drugs and related science required for the treatments. To this day, we have always felt we were receiving the ultimate in care at every turn.

Mid-October of 2014 brought with it the end of the six hormonal chemotherapy treatments and after several weeks of recuperation a return to Dr. Q for a follow up scan. As the mid-term results were very encouraging showing a dramatic reduction in cancer cells and the rehabilitation of bone density, our optimism was showing, our faith was strong but offset with a tempered level of realism. The test results obtained the following day were that of excitement and joy. Sharon's anxiety immediately went from worry to elation and normal breathing when the scans were examined on the computer monitor and virtually all of the cancer cells discovered in the previous tests were gone.

The ribs, lymph nodes, spinal lesions, and the 100% infected sacrum were clear of cancer and the lost bone density had been replaced with healthy new calcium deposits. We were blown away by what we were viewing and being witness to, the power of God and the wisdom that had been bestowed upon my entire medical team to date.

"To say the least, we were ecstatic as God had just delivered our Miracle in life!"

To say the least, we were ecstatic as God had just delivered our miracle in life!   A sidebar to the extraordinary positive results is that on the day we received the good news we had an unusually long wait to see Dr. Q. Normally waits are measured in minutes but today it was two or three hours. We surmised later that he had many appointments with patients that day and much of it delivering less than pleasant news to many. I believe my test results and the positive discussion of them made the Doctor's day, he was able to end on a positive note and consequently, we had little problem with the wait. We prayed for those patients and families that came before us and could not wait to begin our trip back north and home.

We were so pleased with the results that a few weeks later Sharon, being the thoughtful person she is and knowing full well that for the last fifty or so years I had been yearning to buy a sports car as I had a '62 roadster prior to our marriage. She suggested that to celebrate the event even beyond the blessing that God had bestowed on us, that we should buy another and I would be whole again.

Of course, I had little argument with this suggestion and coyly and quietly agreed that this might be a good idea. I am a practical 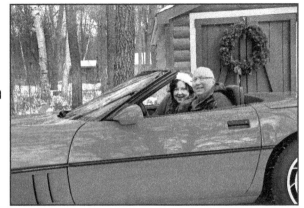 person when it comes to spending dollars needlessly and suggested that we search for a used Corvette™ and a number of years of age to keep the cost to a minimum as this may turn out to be just a lark.

I searched the online lists of cars and found a 1987 red convertible with 33,000 actual miles located in Denver for $6500. Our son Marc happened to live in the Denver area and he made a trip to the car's location the following Saturday and gave it his blessing as he is also a "car guy". We purchased it and made arrangements to have it delivered to our home in Brainerd. It arrived about a week later, my dreams had come true and to this day it is still sitting in our garage waiting for pleasant side trips under God's sky.

What a wonderful wife and life!

"The Good News and the Bad"

Chapter 7

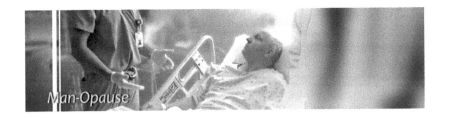

Man-Opause

It seems that all of life is a series of good news-bad news days. The new word in our vocabulary was now a drug by the name of Zytiga™. In the long run, this was really not bad news as it was very effective at heading off some very smart and adaptive prostate cancer cells. In the short run, it was devastating news when Dr. Q gave his explanation of the workings of the drug and laid the cost on us of $8065 per month and required taking it daily for 13 months. When you do the math, this is a lot of money. I was to start the drug in December when I returned for my last monthly injection of the hormone Firmagon ᵗᵐ but time would be needed to make the insurance and financial arrangements.

The prostate cancer cell is very adaptive in that it requires a supply of testosterone to continue to thrive, divide and conquer. Hormone therapy is designed to eliminate the body's ability to produce testosterone thereby starving the cells. Prostate Cancer cells evolve with the unique ability to create their own version of synthetic testosterone and thus continue to thrive often resulting in hormone therapy being a limited means of treating cancer.

This to me was an unbelievable turn of events. As it turns out, Zytiga™ was developed and designed to eliminate this backdoor production of synthetic androgen levels (testosterone) by the cancer cells and once again allow the hormone therapy to do its work. A very small market for a very useful and effective drug, thus the resultant high cost. Struggling to cover the cost of drug treatment such as this became an urgent problem for us. Does Medicare cover this? Does my supplement insurance cover this? How much of the cost am I able to cover personally? What happens if these questions have less than positive answers? How have my odds of beating this cancer changed? These are all very important questions which required an early resolution.

Medicare insurance options have very limited windows for making changes in plans and December was it. Upon arriving back in Brainerd, I was explaining this predicament to a close friend and he suggested I call and visit with a local medical insurance expert and broker that he knew and trusted. They agreed to make time very quickly to meet with Sharon and me regarding this dilemma and we discussed in detail our existing insurance plans and my drug needs. They put their people to work investigating our existing insurance and drug plans and their willingness to cover the new drug costs whether full or partial and Medicare involvement. It was determined that our present medical and drug plans more than likely would not be a good fit for working with the clinics involved and that a switch to other plans was being recommended.

When deciding on coverage with Medicare plans there is a bit of a crap shoot going on as the individual must make their choice of plans prior to the first of the year and the actual contracts of the insurance companies with Medicare are not final until after the first of the year. This made us somewhat nervous but our consultant covered all of the bases and we needed to continue to move ahead. The switch in plans was made at that point. The identity of the insurance companies and plans are not of importance to this writing but the fact that research and planning are required at every step in fighting this cancer and living life effectively. In Chapter 4 we discussed gambling with decisions regarding your health and life in general and with insurance, this is also the case. We found that Medicare indeed would cover a percentage of the Zytiga™ and our new drug plan would probably also do the same but we were still being left with a co-pay of approximately $2600 per month, still, a staggering amount to contend with.

Life was about to become quite different for us from a financial standpoint. If the results of partial coverage by both Medicare and our drug plan had been negative, we would have had no choice but to decline the use of the drug and our odds would be forever changed of beating cancer. To make a long story short a medical charitable foundation came through in a big way and after reviewing our personal inability to meet the obligation agreed to contribute to the co-pay amounts.

".....Waging a war on cancer can bring financial ruin ....."

We prayed hard to find a solution to the problem, were answered and we will be forever grateful. Our insurance consultant Brian Sedlachek, Central Choice Financial of

Baxter, Minnesota gave us his all is and our hat is off to him and his staff.

We have been blessed by God and to date have fared well financially but for many, waging war on cancer can bring financial ruin and having a handle on your money as well as cancer will be extremely important. Do your homework relating to your insurance and policy coverage prior to beginning treatment as well as research into other available funding will pay off in the end.

In March of 2015, we returned for my regular 3-month interval scan, PSA testing and beginning of our newly prescribed oral drug. It must be taken in the early morning hours with no food for at least two hours prior and at least one hour after taking it. I quickly established a routine of waking at 6:00 am every morning, swallow the pills and go back to bed for a couple of hours. The drug was delivered monthly via overnight delivery from the pharmacy and required refrigeration.

The dosage was four 250 mg very large pills per day all taken together. I found that 6 am worked just fine. An oral steroid was prescribed twice daily at 5 mg while on Zytiga™ to reduce fluid retention, hypertension, low potassium blood level, and fatigue, all side effects of the drug. This treatment has been shown through trial and practice to be highly beneficial in the fight against prostate cancer and prolonging life. In retrospect, this demonstrates the vigorous and progressive actions against this disease by my medical team.

Newly discovered drugs that have been of benefit to my fight and other forms of cancer today can be summed up in a quote from the book, Promoting Wellness Beyond Hormone Therapy, Second Edition by Mark A. Moyad, MD, MPH;

"As a patient, knowing about all your options, educating yourself about cancer and working with your doctor can open up many new avenues for you to gain access to other future effective drug treatments."

Coincidentally with the Zytiga™ treatment, hormonal therapy Lupron™ injections at quarterly intervals began in January of 2015 and continued for the next two years in an effort to keep my natural testosterone levels as low as possible. As treatment continued through the year, liver function blood tests were taken regularly to monitor adverse reactions, if any.

Sharon and I needed a break and to get away for some relaxation and mellowing out time. We left on a needed road trip in the fall of 2015 to again visit our son Marc in Denver, CO.   We scheduled it to begin early October and planned to return to Minnesota to meet a regularly scheduled examination and scan on October 29th. By this time we were getting used to seeing positive results from the testing over the last couple of years and we both felt this would be the case again on our return visit. The continued development and accuracy of the scan testing has been advancing and refined quickly in the last few years. When I was beginning my treatment the test was not being given without elevated PSA scores to assure a higher degree of accuracy in the testing. The result of my current October 29th PSA testing was zero, consistent with recent past experience. The scan, however, revealed the possibility of a small malignant tumor in my lower pelvic area and the test results were referred to radiologists for additional study and we met with them on October 30th.

The world turns very quickly when you are in the fight of your life and this was no exception. The discussion with the head of radiation oncology therapy was set for the same day. This included possible general radiation treatment of the pelvic tumor as well as targeted radiation of the previously treated bone cancer lesions. This was to insure that the cancer located at ribs; spine and sacrum locations were permanently eliminated. A study of my radiation therapy records from the 2012 treatment by Dr. Roberts in Brainerd was required by the radiologists to assure that multiple radiation treatments in the same general area were possible.

The records were ordered and later that week they called with an appointment for November 10th to return for "Simulation". In effect, this was a full day of preparation of a body mold and tattoos for reference alignment purposes for testing, contrast CT scan and ultrasound scans to plan for the coming radiation treatments. Nice conclusion to a great fall trip!

Our cat, "Little Guy", tipped the scales at about 17 pounds and after 16 plus years with him, he had become ill about a year and a half prior to the start of this radiation therapy. Our only humane choice was to put him to sleep. This became a very hard time for us as he had become an integral part of our home and lives. It was very hard to think of replacing him and simply was not in the cards until the latest recurrence of cancer.

On our drive home to Nisswa on October 30th, we stopped at an animal shelter in St. Cloud to see what they had in stock, so to speak. We both became somewhat smitten with a three-year-old male with three legs, which of course we would have renamed "Tripod", "Lucky" or something similar. We were just shopping that day and decided to sleep on it and continued our journey north. Twenty-four hours later, we had decided to return to the shelter and adopt Tripod and make him a part of our lives and family. We were disappointed for ourselves but happy for him to find another loving family had beaten us to him.

As we scanned the fifty or so remaining cats, a black and white Tuxedo shorthair with very cool facial markings caught our eye and he was placed in my arms by the attendant - it was destiny.

Seven months of cool and love, he snuggled and purred his way into our hearts and today Rizzo is a very important part of life in the Harris household. Animals can be very therapeutic in times of healing and stress and are recommended to all.

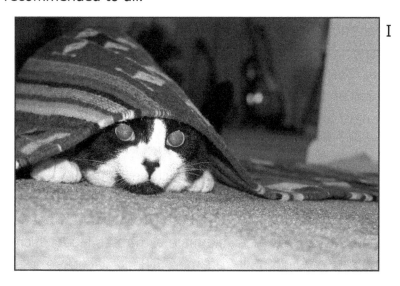

I throw this into the mix because as fate would have it, confirmation of the existence of the malignant prostate cancer tumor in my pelvic area did not occur until after the 30th. Now we have a growing kitten in a strange new home and within two weeks we will be living away from Sunday evening through Friday evening every week until Christmas. We are fortunate to have wonderful friends and neighbors who stepped up to the plate and visited multiple times daily while we were gone and made sure that Rizzo was loved and cared for properly while our lives were temporarily turned upside down.

He may have been wondering what kind of crazy life was traded for his cozy home in the shelter but he adapted quickly and is loved by all.

God is good and so are rescue cats.

"Simulation Day"

Chapter 8

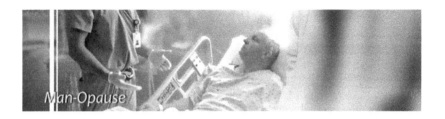

Simulation day was one which has been very hard to forget. It began at 7:30 AM in radiation therapy where we were immediately referred back to urology to have my old and dear friend, the Foley catheter inserted so that contrast could be introduced to my bladder for the scans and ultrasound testing later when I returned to radiation.

Now, this was to be a temporary situation mind you, a catheter for a day to facilitate the scheduled tests. Two nurses and a 30 year veteran of catheter insertion and the clinic resident expert, failed at several attempts to successfully insert a catheter due to a blockage in the urethra at the bladder. I was then sent to a scoping examination room to be examined by a urologist utilizing a flexible cystoscope to view the obstruction. I was one of five in the room watching in living color on a monitor when it was discovered that it was scar tissue as a result of my radiation treatments in 2012 in Brainerd.

I asked at the time if this was a major problem and the doctor *"Sounds easy but ...."* replied that it was going to be solved by inserting a wire through the cystoscope and open the obstruction. Sounds easy but imagine the amount of discomfort I was already in after four attempts to insert a catheter and now have a roomful of doctors and assistants carving their way to my bladder through a tube. Success was had as promised, however, and "Foley" was once again installed and a part of me. Unfortunately, this was just the beginning of a long day and an hour or so after entering urology I limped back to the waiting room and a very concerned wife.

As we left the waiting area I noticed a number of men and a few ladies now becoming agitated and visibly concerned as to what will happen to them when their turn came. They watched me hobble daintily past and began the long trek back to the radiation therapy folks. My reward for all of this early morning activity was that I got to keep "Foley" for another week instead of just the day, in order for the impromptu surgery to heal and then have to learn to relieve myself all over again.   It felt like an old home week.

Due to the time lost in urology inserting the catheter, Sharon and I were running late getting to the scheduled scans and body positioning casting in the radiation therapy department so we began the trek back as quickly as possible. This was not a jog, however, as I was somewhat constrained by my new friend hanging out of me, a urine bag strapped to my ankle and I was very sore. The CT scan and ultrasound testing were time-consuming and intense and I was filled with contrast in my bladder, rectum, and spine. I was immobilized to a point of no movement at all for close to 45 painful minutes in a large tube while the scans were performed. This was for the determination of very precise locations of my internal structure to assure successful radiation therapy beginning in a week or so.

All in all, the morning came and went, lunch was skipped and the tasks came to a conclusion after 3 pm. Exhausted, sore and hungry we decided that the best place to get this day behind us and start recuperating was home.   Off we went and a few hours later we were home in Nisswa, some 15 miles north of Brainerd. A very long day indeed had come to an end and Rizzo greeted us enthusiastically.

 A week later, my close friend Gary Hasse (not to be confused with Gary Harris) accompanied me on a one day drive down and back to the clinic to have "Foley" removed and hopefully be able to void my bladder with little fanfare. We are very good friends and the long day gave us a great opportunity to bond over many common areas of interest. I checked in at urology and when the nurse came to my exam room she informed me that the urologist that performed the blockage removal had left an order that I was to keep "Foley" until I returned in a week or so to begin the scheduled radiation treatments.

Not a happy camper after a long drive to have "Foley" removed, I insisted that it happen now and I will take my chances. Several minutes later the order was changed and the catheter was removed with instructions not to leave the clinic until I was able to void myself without trouble. After a nervous lunch and a lot of water, it worked and off we went back to Brainerd and "Foley" was once again in the wastebasket. Rest stops were, however, a unique pleasure and frequent on the return trip.

As I look back, the whole experience of removal of the blockage turned out to be a blessing in disguise as my passing of water was becoming increasingly difficult with time and the procedure has solved the problem to date. You might say that for every door that closes, another sphincter opens.

"New Friends & the Hope Lodge"

Chapter 9

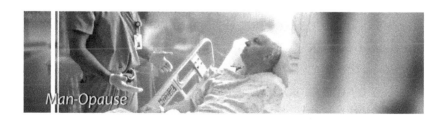

The third week of November 2015 brought with it the start of radiation therapy for both the newfound pelvic tumor and the targeted radiation of the bone cancer areas treated by chemotherapy the year before. This was meant to deliver the coup d'état to the cancer lesions that once existed.

The routine was a daily visit to radiation therapy which meant of course that being away from home we had to make living arrangements for Sunday through Thursday nights. There were many options and We opted for a suites hotel located near the clinic which gave us the ability to easily walk to the appointments. This was somewhat expensive when you

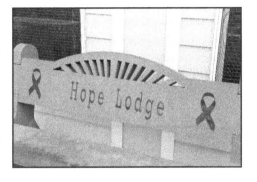

combined the lodging with all of your meals being out but only a temporary solution until the Hope Lodge™, owned and operated by the American Cancer Society™, opened its welcome doors to us.

The waiting period to being accepted was approximately ten days from the start of the radiation therapy and being placed in the queue for this was an automated process initiated by the clinic on our behalf once they had established my radiation schedules. We were continually being reminded that between God and the medical team, we were in great hands. The "Lodge" was a Godsend, located near clinics and is operated without charge for 60 patients and a caregiver for each currently undergoing treatment for cancer.

Comfortable hotel style rooms with walk-in bath are standard and assignments of refrigerator and kitchen cabinet space are made to each resident in one of several kitchens. There are five different common kitchen and dining areas as well as several living rooms with large screen television, couches and chairs for residents to mingle, meet and create new and often lasting friendships. Normally, you prepare your own meals and do kitchen patrol but a wonderful side benefit during the Christmas weeks is that organizations from around the area including schools, businesses, and fraternal groups have planned evenings with meals and programs for all.

It took us only a day or so until we met and made new friends and began to share our cancer treatment stories, mutual interests and minister to each other. Many are in dire straits and depressed when they check in. We became a part of amazing changes in self-confidence and the will to beat their cancers as we were all sharing a common fight for life. Being able to minister to and receive support from others was a life-changing experience for both of us and quite likely for the vast majority of our new "family".

The standard radiation treatment consists of thirty-three daily treatments, with the exception of holidays and weekends. Chemotherapy normally consists of six infusions spaced three weeks apart. Residents are allowed to remain at the Hope Lodge for the duration of their treatment and then leave for home. Accordingly, some are there for only a few weeks and others for months at a time but the relationships are every bit as strong.

Our stay began the last week in November and continued through my last radiation treatment which was Christmas Eve day. We discovered a bonus in that this was a wonderful time of the year to be a part of the group ministry as the Christmas season is a time of extraordinary outpourings of love and concern from the community. Two or three times a week during our stay, school groups, businesses, and other organizations provided home cooked and served meals to all and gifts of Christmas treats were delivered to the Hope Lodge tm on a daily basis providing a touch of home and a bond for us to relax, share experiences and provide ministry and support to each other.

Mike, a postal employee from Iowa, was undergoing radiation treatment for his initial bout with prostate cancer and became a fast friend as we shared a common interest in our health and with daily games of cribbage both individually and with others in team play. This was also in the heart of football season with collegiate and professional teams providing spirited discussions from opposing camps of fans. There was an equal number of Packer and Viking fans living at the Lodge and they can be as loyal and combative as liberals and conservatives.

This was a humbling experience as we were introduced to men, women, young adults and seniors with cancer conditions that seemed insurmountable in comparison to my own. A forty-something young woman was fighting esophageal cancer and had her stomach and esophagus removed with an entirely new system constructed from her upper colon. This surprisingly was not an uncommon condition and surgical procedure. She was accompanied as caregivers by her young adult son and daughter that rotated their residence to care for their mother. Adding to the distress, she had a younger child at home in northern Minnesota and she too traveled on weekends for that taste of home helping to sustain a positive motivation. She was a passionate woman and close to her God giving her a level of resolve which was inspiring to us all. She was an example of a large number of the sixty residents that were on the edge of life but were inspired by the positive atmosphere of nearly 120 others around them that were now their new families.

There were those when they first arrived, spoke of their cancer as being terminal with only a few days or weeks remaining. Due to the spirit found in this great place, the love of the people around them and the opportunity to share a common faith in God their lives forever changed and most went on to live much longer lives than they thought possible.

Both Sharon and I are driven by doing what we can to share our talents and enthusiasm with others, especially those in need of a friend, love and moral support. Since retirement some ten years hence, my life-long passion and hobby in photography have grown to that of professional

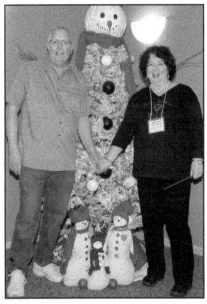

or at the very least semi-professional level. I explained this to the staff of the Hope Lodge™ two weeks before Christmas and enlisted their blessing and support to provide photographs to the residents and their caregivers by one of the six beautiful Christmas trees that adorned the home in the lounges, dining areas, and living rooms.

"... this may provide a positive memory ..."

We proposed to take photographs of those that wished to participate, by the tree of their choice and we would provide prints, enlargements and digital files, provided without charge and with our love. Nothing like this had been attempted in the past as far as we knew, and dealing with people that are fighting for their lives, we hoped this may provide a positive memory of their time in cancer treatment.

The staff created a flyer that was distributed to all of the residents and listed the times and date of the photography and then we waited for a response. The turnout was gratifying as over 60% responded and they showed up with bells on, so to speak, for their chance at a pleasant moment during these monumental times in their lives.

All of the photography was completed in one day and we brought the digital images back to our Nisswa home that Friday evening when our treatment week was completed. I spent most of that weekend at the computer and printer processing the images and it was a labor of love looking at the beaming faces that now had hope, at least for a brief moment in time. We completed the task and enveloped and labeled each package of love that we brought back to our "home" the following Sunday evening.

Monday was a thrilling and very pleasant day for us as so many of our new family now had their Christmas memory of themselves and their caregiver to cherish into the future. All in all, this was a success, a blessing to us and smiles all around.

During the entire seven weeks of radiation therapy we commuted every week for a total of some 3200 miles and God smiled on us. The entire time the roads were great and Minnesota winter held off until just the week after Christmas when the snow and cold settled in.

Again we were blessed.

"Graduation Day"

Chapter 10

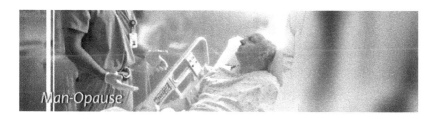

Man-Opause

On Christmas Eve day, 2015 my last of the thirty-three radiation sessions was completed at 11:30 am and it was my honor to ring the bell of success in the radiation therapy lounge, being a graduation day tradition.

After standard radiation to eliminate the pelvic cancer tumor and five high-dose targeted radiation applications

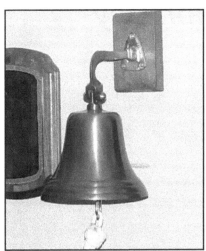

to my previous bone cancer lesions, it indeed was graduation and after ringing the bell we were on our way back home to a relatively normal existence once again. As a bonus, we were excited to welcome little Rizzo to our family on a full-time basis and we were among the last to pack and check out of the Hope Lodge™ which left saying "*goodbye*" to be a bittersweet moment.

Daughter Joy and son Marc normally visit for the Christmas holiday and they were joining us once again this year to welcome our time of cheer. As we knew exactly what our schedule was going to be, they arranged their flights from California and Colorado to arrive on the afternoon of December 24th to coincide with our travels back home to Nisswa. We met up with them at the Minneapolis airport terminals and headed north.

A long-standing tradition in our family is attending church service on Christmas Eve and as we were in the twin cities we altered the route and paid a visit to our old church congregation in Burnsville and arrived just in time to catch their Christmas celebration. It was very inspiring and therapeutic for us.

Christmas Eve is one of those few times of the year when you find your choices for dining out next to impossible. We were passing the north edge of the Twin Cities when we opted for Christmas Eve dinner at a large chain restaurant. This was less than a great experience but provided us with the opportunity for an in-depth discussion on the trip home to evaluate the best and worst of our many Christmas Eve dinners together.

Sharon is a Christmas junky that decorates our home from thirty or so stored boxes of decorations and love over a period of five weeks prior to Christmas. Not to be outdone, I light up the yard with several hundred lights to add to the festive atmosphere of our home and neighborhood.

Due to our schedule for the previous seven weeks or so in treatment, the decorating fetish did not occur and our welcome home was somewhat diminished. We celebrate the holidays each year with a few very close friends and relatives and this year was going to be no different. Knowing we would be home by Christmas day, the invitations had gone out to Sharon's Sister Jan and husband Jack from Bemidji, the Craguns from Brainerd, Dave an old and close friend of Joy, Sharon's cousin David and wife Bine and a couple of neighbors to join us on December 26th and 27th. Of course, we had little to feed these people and Sharon needed the 25th to scratch her decorating itch.

Those that are close to you are of prime importance when you are in a battle for your life and again this was demonstrated with Sister Jan insisting on preparing the Christmas meal for all. What a beautiful and heartfelt gesture of love on their part as well as the houseful of guests adding the personal support, necessary trimmings and gifts to fill out the two days of love and celebration.

This turned into a very blessed Christmas for us after all.

"Scan-xiety & the Road Ahead"

epilogue

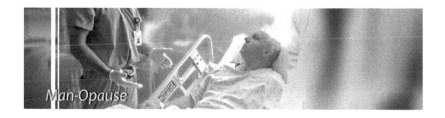

Man-Opause My Continuing Battle with Metastatic Prostate Cancer

The foregoing discussion of my trials, tears, elation, and triumphs over recurrent metastatic prostate cancer has been written beginning in early 2018 in the hope and faith that our battle will continue to be successful in the coming months and years. To date, I have beaten the odds due to our faith in God, a team of medical professionals that have cared deeply about delivering their top service, motivation to remain positive in the face of great adversity, and family and friends that have always been there for us.

Over the last ten years I have undergone surgery for a radical prostatectomy to remove a cancerous prostate along with thirteen lymph nodes; radiation treatment for a recurrent prostate cancer tumor adjacent to my bladder; chemohormonal therapy for recurrent prostate cancer lesions in two ribs, two locations in my spine and my sacrum; radiation therapy for a recurrent prostate cancer tumor in my lower pelvic area; targeted high dose radiation therapy in all of the bone lesion areas previously treated with chemotherapy; and some twenty plus scans, most of which were within the last eight years.

The common term used with the scans in the fight on cancer is "scan-xiety" which simply means that with every scan there is accompanying wait and stress as the results are being delivered. If you have one or twenty, this is always the case and depression may not be far behind. My scans continue to this day on at least a six-month basis and "scan-xiety" is still a part of our lives.

The beginning of this journey was a simple but effective physical examination of the prostate gland in a very normal annual checkup with my family practice physician. I owe him my life as without his diligence and professionalism I would not have taken the timely steps I did to wage war with my cancer. Several years before my diagnosis, he also discovered Sharon's kidney cancer at an early stage and set in motion her remission. I believe God placed Dr. Nordahl in our world to save our lives for a definite future purpose.

We have been fortunate and blessed to know and have the services and friendship of one of the top urologic surgeons in the country Dr. Mark Fallen, who also successfully cared for Sharon with her kidney cancer. Upon providing the expert surgery and follow up services possible at the onset of my prostate cancer, he had the contacts and where with all to refer me to a friend and colleague in a separate clinic where I believe I found the most advanced diagnostic and recurrent prostate cancer treatment in the world today. My personal physician Dr.

"My winning battle with prostate cancer was one of being in the right place at the right time, ..."

James Freeman has provided close cover for me over the ten years I have been in the lake country. Jim was the one I turned to for my prostate cancer pre-surgery physical ten years ago and he has been there for me watching over my general health and well being as I have waged this war on cancer and it on me.

My winning battle with prostate cancer was one of being in the right place at the right time, having the fortune to be in the presence of the best medical professionals, the best wife and caregiver, loving family, wonderful and caring friends, terrific church family and blessed with the hand of God always resting on our shoulders.

Last March on my 76th birthday our daughter Joy posted on her social media page an unexpected tribute to me wherein she recited the number of times to date that I had fought cancer and been victorious where she stated that I am a *"warrior"*. Indeed I feel like a warrior and recommend this positive attitude for the reader as well.

Homework and research are essential in any fight if you expect to be victorious. The more you know about your enemy, in this case prostate cancer, the better equipped you will be to select your medical team, to remain positive, to inspire those around you and to be confident that your choices are correct. It is my hope and prayer that you will take away from this account of my experiences a reference to make better choices than those of the uninformed. Having an awareness of my successes and possible mistakes in timing and selection of treatments, your chances of victory will hopefully be inhanced in the end.

I understand there is no cure for metastatic prostate cancer at the present time other than early discovery and removal of the prostate prior to metastasis. The fight we wage is simply to continue living and be in control by staying abreast of all of the new technological breakthroughs in disease control and diagnosis. A permanent cure will be found one day and we will be ready. Assemble your pieces of the prostate cancer puzzle with regular physical examinations and PSA testing from a knowledgeable team. Diagnosis at the onset of prostate cancer and of recurrent prostate cancers once they have become metastatic will provide the opportunity for early treatment and will allow you to function in a relatively normal lifestyle well into the future.

I recently read that as of 2018, the U.S. Preventative Services Task Force suggests that men over 70 years of age could skip the PSA test as prostate cancer is relatively slow growing. However, If you have a father or brother that had prostate cancer at age 65 or earlier advice is to investigate with your doctor to begin testing at age 45.

Medical science has evolved rapidly in the ten years since my struggle began and new methods of diagnosis and treatment are constantly being developed. Today many needle biopsies can be avoided with the utilization of diagnostic exam called a multi-parametric MRI. This can cover the entire prostate gland making it easier to spot malignancies and their severity than with the random tissue sampling of the biopsy. Should the result of the

MRI be positive however, the biopsy may still be required to determine the extent and grading of the suspected prostate cancer.

Recently a new treatment for prostate and other cancers is being utilized involving the use of ablation which is a probe inserted into the patient that is computer targeted exactly on the cancer cell and utilizes heat, super cold (cryoblation), radio frequency or high intensity focused ultra sound to kill the cancer cell. Ablation has been used for years in the treatment of certain heart disease and to our benefit has been expanded to the treatment of cancers. These are only examples of the rapid developments in the fight of cancers and you are encouraged to research and investigate these and all other means of fighting your disease. An informed patient is a winning patient.

"An informed patient is a winning patient."

My heart goes out to cancer victims that are left to fight the battle alone as care givers are God's blessing to us. Cancer and the fight that is waged with it may very well be more difficult on those around the patient than the patient. It is so difficult to be near yet so far as your caregiver will want in the worst way to provide aid in any physical way possible and to provide needed moral support. What an important role to play! I could feel Sharon's pain daily when my skirmishes were being waged and her frustration at not having a switch to simply turn off my anxiety, pain, and discomfort. Love is a magnificent thing and grows stronger as times become more difficult.

As a cancer fighter and survivor, you do not need to be alone. Ask those around you for support and try to have a friendship circle that seems never-ending.

"Lean on a number of very close friends ...."

Lean on a number of very close friends that you can, like me, know are always there when we require physical assistance or a morale boost. I only have to call and they come. Embrace and thank God for those around you that lovingly provide for your comfort and healing.

One of society's new buzzwords is "Resilience". This is simply the ability to bounce back from adversity and deal with life's challenges, tribulations and downturns. This is despite the events being totally devastating and overwhelming. You still have the stress in dealing with the events but being able to deal and adapt to the adversity is paramount. We have worked very hard to be resilient and positive and to this day remain so.

I have been blessed to be on the receiving end of amazing technology, brilliant professionals utilizing new curative measures, my receipt of heavenly miracles and to now have the opportunity to pay it forward by providing a helping hand to others that are in need of information and a friend.

In conclusion, we all have something to offer from our life experiences, accumulation of knowledge and contacts made. It is my goal that this account of my cancer experiences may help you defeat your enemy, and build a lasting and trusting friendship between myself and the reader.

Gary Harris

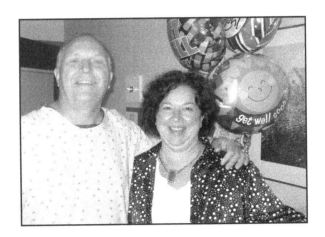

"Come to Me all who are weary and carrying heavy burdens and I will give you rest. Take My yoke upon you and Learn from Me for I am gentle and humble in heart, and you will find rest for your souls."

Mathew 11:28-30

CPSIA information can be obtained
at www.ICGtesting.com
Printed in the USA
FSHW020036071119
63827FS

9 780578 540641